SWALLOWING GUIDELINES

Individualised Programmes of Care

SWALLOWING GUIDELINES

Individualised Programmes of Care

Elizabeth Boaden & Jo Walker

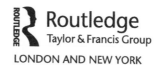

Routledge
Taylor & Francis Group

LONDON AND NEW YORK

First published 2005 by Speechmark Publishing Ltd.

Published 2017 by Routledge
2 Park Square, Milton Park, Abingdon, Oxon OX14 4RN
711 Third Avenue, New York, NY 10017, USA

Routledge is an imprint of the Taylor & Francis Group, an informa business

British Library Cataloguing in Publication Data
Boaden, Elizabeth
    Swallowing guidelines : individualised programmes of care
    1. Deglutition disorders – Treatment
    I. Title   II. Walker, Jo
    616.3'206

ISBN-13: 9780863885174 (pbk)

CONTENTS

ACKNOWLEDGEMENTS

The authors would like to express their thanks to: Deirdre Rainbow, Principal Speech and Language Therapist in Adult Neurology; Jo Marks, Specialist Speech and Language Therapist in Paediatric Dysphagia; and Chris Airey, IT Director, for their invaluable critiques, enthusiasm and expertise, without which this work would not have been possible.

Thank you.

Supplementary Resources Disclaimer

Additional resources were previously made available for this title on CD. However, as CD has become a less accessible format, all resources have been moved to a more convenient online download option.

You can find these resources available here: http://resourcecentre.routledge.com/books/9780863885174

Please note: Where this title mentions the associated disc, please use the downloadable resources instead.

INTRODUCTION

This UK-devised resource allows you to produce multiple individual dysphagia programmes that may be emailed or posted to individuals, their carers (parents are included in the use of this term) or other professionals, in any location. As there is considerable overlap of information, advice and therapy between client groups, this resource is a collated, accessible menu that takes a holistic approach to dysphagia management of all client groups.

This flexible resource enables you to design contemporaneous written information, advice, therapy, diary sheets to record oral intake and feeding behaviour, stickers for drug charts, and swallowing guideline signs for any setting, all of which are personalised to you and your department. It describes all aspects of dysphagia care in a clear, logical, jargon-free format. The format reflects a time-line of considerations, from pre-feeding stimulation, environment and posture, to equipment, food or drink consistencies and specific swallowing techniques. Additional sections serve as aides-memoires to ensure that all aspects of management are considered. The resource also offers an introduction to swallowing dysfunction, promoting a framework in which to incorporate accepted clinical practice. It allows you to insert and select specific advice from highlighted sections or add to the free text boxes to allow maximum individualisation. The programme may be amended quickly as individual status changes. Consequently, the individual may have updated programmes according to their stage of ability as they progress through dysphagia management. This provides a route to map clinical outcomes.

The disk and accompanying template ensures that individual dysphagia programmes are comprehensive and produced efficiently, thus maximising use of clinical and administrative time. The template is a numbered list indicating all the information available in the resource. The highlighted choices and free text boxes are also indicated to enable you to identify quickly the information you wish to be included in the programme. Once the template is complete, the information can be selected immediately from the disk copy and within a few minutes you will have produced an individual dysphagia management programme that is ready to be emailed or posted (see examples in the appendices).

All staff, including any new or bank staff or students, and carers, need to be aware of the swallowing recommendations.

It is important to be aware of the literature about carer and patient non-compliance with written guidelines (Chadwick *et al*, 2002). Therefore therapists should continue to give verbal descriptions and modelling of swallowing advice as well as the rationale and expected outcomes. If some carers are more able to undertake practical feeding techniques or supervisory roles, it is important that they are identified in the programme. To encourage compliance further, diagrams have also been used in the resource. Therapists should agree guidelines with clients and carers, and ensure that review dates are set.

This resource does not give academic advice, nor is it an alternative to current best practice.

HOW TO USE THIS RESOURCE

- Make a copy of the Template from the book.

- Using the Manual for reference, circle the corresponding numbers on the Template. Indicate relevant diagrams and choices within the options for each statement and write in any additional information where indicated.

- Once the template has been completed, the information can be put onto the CD-ROM to create a personalised set of guidelines.

- The CD-ROM will normally auto-start – simply place the CD in your drive and wait for the programme to start. It is always recommended to close down other applications beforehand. If auto-start is disabled on your PC, then you will need to run the file Swallowing.exe, which can be found in the root folder of the CD.

- Click on the 'Template' icon to begin creating the document.

- Complete the personal information and select the file location to save the document on your computer.

- Use the 'Next' buttons to move from one page to the next. You can go back at any time by using the 'Back' buttons.

- Click on the relevant numbers on each page, highlighting any required diagrams and choosing from the drop-down options as appropriate.

- Complete any blank boxes where necessary, for example to specify frequency.

- Add any additional information in the 'Comments' box at the end of each section.

- Select any additional resources required, such as diary sheets. A sign or notice can be created showing requirements for food, fluid and position by selecting the appropriate diagrams. The diary sheets and recording sheets are also available as PDFs in the 'Resources' section of the program.

- The Guidelines will be saved when you click 'Next' on the final screen. They can then be printed out or sent by e-mail.

- Please note that Microsoft Word must be installed on your PC in order to create personalised guidelines. Also, Adobe Acrobat Reader is required to view the documents in the Resources section and if you do not have this, it can be downloaded free of charge from the Adobe website at www.adobe.com.

MANUAL
FOR SWALLOWING
GUIDELINES

- Identify from the manual the statements and information applicable to the individual.

- Then circle the corresponding numbered statements and information on the template to be included in the final programme and put a line through items or information to be deleted.

- Take care to write in specific additional information where indicated on the template.

SWALLOWING GUIDELINES

WRITTEN BY _____ DATE _____

NAME _____ DOB _____

Routledge
Taylor & Francis Group
ROUTLEDGE

DESCRIPTION OF SWALLOWING DIFFICULTIES

1 The throat muscles are not coordinating properly. This means that rather than food or drink going down your throat to the stomach, there is a risk of it going into the lungs. This is called 'aspiration'.

2 The throat muscles that squeeze food and drink into the food pipe are weak. This causes food or drink either to stick or to move more slowly down the throat. This can be uncomfortable and can cause further problems if there is food residue left in the throat.

3 The muscle in your throat, which opens and closes to control how and when food and drink are pushed down towards your stomach, is not opening in the right way and at the right time. Food and drink may enter the lungs instead of going down into the stomach. It may also cause a sticking sensation and may take many swallows to get a very small quantity of food and drink down. This can be extremely tiring.

4 Because the muscles in the mouth (eg, tongue, cheeks, lips, jaw) are weak, it may be difficult to move food around the mouth without getting it lodged between the teeth and cheeks. It may also be difficult to chew or prevent food and drink escaping from the lips. This can make mealtimes very tiring and problematic.

5 The messages being sent to and from the muscles of the mouth via the brain are damaged. Consequently, the mouth is not always able to detect that food or drink is present and needs to be swallowed. Overlarge bites may be taken, or food may stay in the mouth or be spat out.

6 The messages being sent to and from the muscles in the mouth via the brain are damaged, causing the mouth to move in an uncoordinated or different way. It may be difficult to get food and drink into the mouth. Once it is in the mouth, the food and drink may then be difficult to control and may not be swallowed safely.

7 Coughing is your body's natural way of removing material from your windpipe and is at times normal.

8 Before starting a meal or drink, ensure there is someone near who has the prerequisite training or knowledge to recognise when someone is choking and is able to perform the necessary techniques to remove the obstruction.

9 When something does 'go down the wrong way' and into the lungs, this is called 'aspiration'. Signs of aspiration are: excessive or frequent coughing; wet, gargly voice quality; change in breathing rate; change in colour; recurrent chest infections. If aspiration occurs frequently it can cause chronic

Routledge
Taylor & Francis Group

chest infections and problems. This may mean that you need to: [do exercises to strengthen muscles needed for swallowing]; [practice how to swallow in a different way]; [alter the way you swallow]; [change the textures of what you eat and/or drink]. It is important to follow the guidelines below to prevent or reduce the severity of the swallowing problem, and to minimise the risk of choking or swallowing things the wrong way. If any difficulties are noted, please check that the advice is being followed, before contacting the person identified on the front of the guidelines.

Comments

ORAL DESENSITISATION EXERCISES

[To be completed ____ times/day.]

1   Support the [lips / jaw] as indicated in the diagrams.

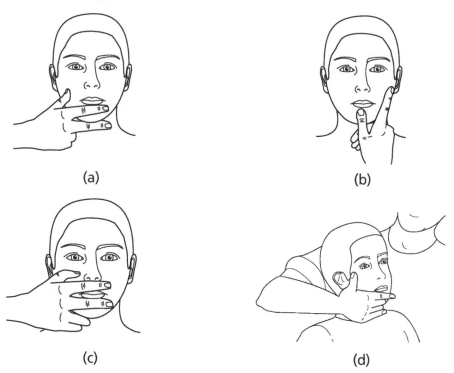

(a)

(b)

(c)

(d)

2   [Gently / firmly] [stroke / pat] the cheeks in preparation for oral desensitisation [and repeat ____ times].

Routledge
Taylor & Francis Group

3   [Gently / firmly] [stroke / pat] the jaw, cheeks and lips and under the chin, working towards the mouth [and repeat ___ times].

4   [Gently / firmly] [stroke / pat] down the sides of the nose towards the upper lip (as indicated on the diagram) [and repeat ___ times].

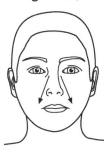

5   Place a [specify], as an oral stimulator, underneath the top lip and slide it firmly and slowly along the upper gum.

Repeat ___ times and then turn the oral stimulator so that the cheek is pushed out slightly.

Pause, then repeat along the lower gum on the same side.

Pause, then move the oral stimulator along gum on the opposite side.

Pause, then move the oral stimulator along lower gum on the same side [and repeat ___ times].

6   [Gently / Firmly] [stroke / pat] the tongue tip with your [specify], as an oral stimulator.

7   [Gently / Firmly] move your [specify], as an oral stimulator, back towards the first third of the tongue [and repeat ___ times].

8   Use a [specify], as an oral stimulator, to press down on the tongue tip. Gradually move the pressure towards the back of the tongue (stop before gagging occurs) and move it forward again. Continue to move forwards and backwards along the tongue with firm pressure rhythmically, in time to music.

9   [Gently / Firmly] place a [specify], as an oral stimulator, on the ridge behind the top teeth to indicate where to place the tongue tip. Repeat ___ times.

10 Encourage oral manipulation of textured objects.

11 Encourage oral manipulation of objects that have been flavoured.

Comments

Routledge
Taylor & Francis Group

INTRODUCTION OF A TOOTHBRUSH INTO THE MOUTH

[To be completed ___ times/day.]

1   Using a [small, soft silicone-bristled brush, which fits on to a little finger / small headed soft toothbrush / normal toothbrush], rub along the outside of the upper and lower gum ridges, the biting surfaces of the teeth and the inside surface of the teeth [and repeat ___ times].

2   Brush the tongue, teeth and lips [and repeat ___ times].

3   Brush the sides of the tongue [and repeat ___ times].

4   Introduce tastes or toothpaste on the brush [and repeat ___ times].

5   Use an electronic toothbrush to introduce vibration into the mouth [and repeat ___ times].

6   Remember positive eating experiences.

> **Comments**
>
>
>
>
>
>

ENVIRONMENT

Note: The environment affects muscle tone and influences individuals' ability to concentrate and to swallow.

1   If it helps, eat in a quiet room without too many distractions. Consider:

   (a) closing the curtains

   (b) dim lighting

   (c) reducing background noise (eg, turn off radio or television)

   (d) moving away from people who are talking or moving around, as this may be distracting

   (e) removing unnecessary things from the dining table (eg, flowers or tissues).

Routledge
Taylor & Francis Group
ROUTLEDGE

2   If it helps, eat in a more stimulating environment. Consider:

(a) quiet, soothing background noise or music

(b) brightly coloured mats or cutlery

(c) sitting in front of a mirror

(d) sitting at a table with others in a small group.

> **Comments**

EQUIPMENT

Note: Special equipment may improve the way in which food and drink is received.

1   Make sure specialised mealtime equipment is used.

2   Remember to use a [napkin / apron] when eating and drinking.

3   For [meals [and] drinks] check that you are using [your / a]:

(a) plate guard

(b) plate [specify]

(c) bowl [specify]

(d) cup [specify]

(e) beaker [specify]

(f) straw [specify]

(g) angled cutlery [specify]

(h) spoon [specify]

(i) teaspoon [specify]

(j) fork [specify]

(k) cutlery [specify]

(l) non-slip mat [specify]

(m) bottle [specify]

(n) teat [specify]

> **Comments**

Routledge
Taylor & Francis Group
ROUTLEDGE

TEXTURES AND CONSISTENCIES

Note: Some consistencies are easier and safer to swallow than others.

1   Your nutritional needs and fluid requirements are being met adequately via the tube. However, you can have [food / drink] for pleasure. Please adhere to the following guidelines for anything taken orally.

Food

2   You are able to have a fully varied diet. There are no foods you need to avoid.

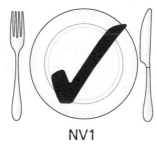

NV1

3   You should have foods that are soft and moist, for example tender meat casseroles (approx 1.5 cm-diced pieces), mashed potato, sponge and custard. Avoid foods:

- of a mixed consistency, such as cereals that do not absorb milk;
- that are hard and dry, such as nuts, pastry and biscuits;
- which have husks, skins or are fibrous, such as sweetcorn, peas, grapes, beans, celery and orange.

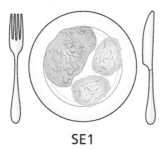

SE1

4   You should have foods that are soft, moist and easy to chew, for example [standard 7-month baby jars – soft and lumpy], Weetabix™, porridge, shepherd's pie, flaked fish in thick sauce, stewed fruit and thick custard.

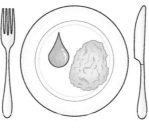

SD1

This page may be photocopied for instructional use only. *Swallowing Guidelines* © Elizabeth Boaden & Jo Walker, 2005

Routledge
Taylor & Francis Group

5   You should have foods that are of a thick, smooth consistency. A blender is an ideal way to achieve this (see manufacturer's instructions). Avoid using water to keep the food moist, as this adds bulk rather than any nutritional value. Add gravy, sauce, cream or milk, for example mousse, thick smooth yoghurt, blended mince and gravy.

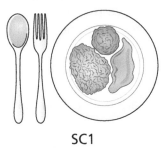

SC1

6   You should have foods that are smooth and moist with a 'drop' consistency. This texture would slip through a fork and needs to be eaten with a spoon, for example [standard 4-month baby jars – smooth purée], thick custard or soft whipped cream.

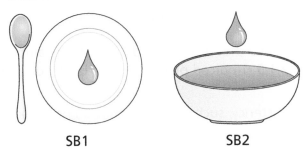

SB1   SB2

7   You should have food with a smooth pouring consistency, which should be eaten with a spoon, such as creamed soup or thin custard.

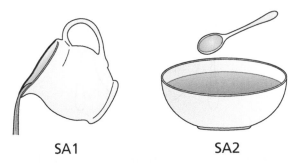

SA1   SA2

8   Foods must be of a hard, dry consistency, for example crackers, pastry or biscuits.

9   Eat finger foods, such as chopped fruit or vegetables [specify other examples].

10 Foods should be highly seasoned and flavourful, for example curry, adding extra herbs and spices.

11 Avoid foods that are difficult to control or move in your mouth, such as jelly, melon or pastes. Opt for semi-solid consistencies, such as mousse, flaked fish in sauce and shepherd's pie.

Routledge
Taylor & Francis Group
ROUTLEDGE

Drink

12 You can have normal drinks, for example tea, coffee, water or squash.

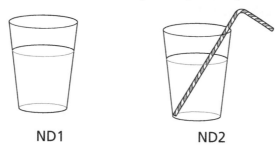

ND1   ND2

13 All food and drinks must be of a thin, watery texture, such as soup or fruit juices.

14 You should have drinks that are naturally thicker in consistency, for example full cream milk, supplement drinks or sip feeds.

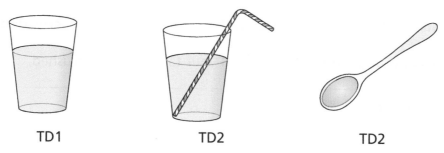

TD1   TD2   TD2

15 Using the thickener prescribed, thicken all thin fluids to a milky consistency. This texture can be drunk through a straw or cup but would leave a thin coating on the back of a spoon (approx ___ scoops of prescribed thickener per 200 ml). Please follow the manufacturer's instructions.

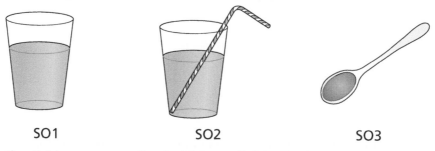

SO1   SO2   SO3

16 Using the thickener prescribed, thicken all thin fluids to a syrup consistency. This texture cannot be drunk through a straw and would leave a thick coating on the back of a spoon (approx ___ scoops of prescribed thickener per 200 ml). Please follow the manufacturer's instructions.

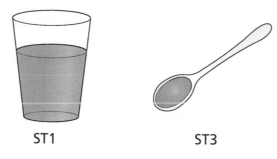

ST1   ST3

This page may be photocopied for instructional use only. *Swallowing Guidelines* © Elizabeth Boaden & Jo Walker, 2005

17 Using the thickener prescribed, thicken all thin fluids to a custard consistency. This texture cannot be drunk through a straw and could only be taken with a spoon (approx ＿ scoops of prescribed thickener per 200 ml). Please follow the manufacturer's instructions.

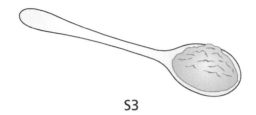

S3

Medication

18 All medication should be taken in syrup or soluble form [and thickened to ＿ consistency].

19 Ensure that all tablets are taken with a drink that is of the specified consistency.

20 Consult your pharmacist to check if your tablets can be crushed.

Comments

GENERAL ADVICE AND PROMPTS

When to eat and drink

Note: The throat muscles may tire at specific times of the day, or during the meal, which may cause aspiration or inadequate nutrition.

1 Rather than having large meals, three times a day, try having smaller more frequent meals [specify].

2 Meals should be spaced out evenly throughout the day.

3 Have each course separately with adequate breaks in between.

4 Since one tires as the day goes on, make sure that you are having a large meal and frequent drinks at the start of the day and just light snacks later.

Routledge
Taylor & Francis Group
ROUTLEDGE

5   Try to eat larger portions when you are feeling at your best.

6   Avoid late evening snacks.

Comments

Preparation

Note: It is important to be comfortable in order to concentrate and to be able to eat and drink as much of the meal as possible.

1   Only eat when you are fully awake and alert.

2   Make sure your glasses are clean, fit securely and are available at mealtimes.

3   Ensure that your hearing aid is working properly and that your ears are clear of wax (so that you will be able to hear any instructions from your carers).

4   If you wear dentures for mealtimes, make sure that they fit and are fixed securely.

Comments

Routledge
Taylor & Francis Group

Tracheostomy Guidelines

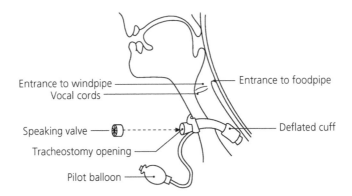

1 Ensure medical or respiratory status is stable for oral intake.

2 Cuff deflation should be tolerated for an appropriate period of time prior to oral intake.

3 Before eating and drinking, ensure that the cuff is deflated before placing the speaking valve.

4 Always check cuff status – do not assume it is deflated.

5 Deflate the cuff fully before any oral intake.

6 Follow the local suction protocol.

7 Keep suction to a minimum.

8 Cover the tracheostomy opening with your thumb or finger only while swallowing. Immediately after each swallow has occurred, take your thumb or finger away to allow a breath out.

9 Monitor secretions suctioned via tracheostomy for food or drink material.

10 Always remove the speaking valve before inflating the cuff.

Comments

Routledge
Taylor & Francis Group

Positioning

Note: Posture affects both muscle tone and the ability to swallow.

1   Use the recommended positioning equipment: that is, standing frame, wedges or wheelchair, etc [and ensure that all the support features are secure, ie_____]

2   Make sure that the height and angle of the chair and table are appropriate.

3   Make sure that you are close enough to the table.

4   You should be able to reach your meal and drink comfortably.

5   Your hips, body, shoulders and head should all be aligned, and you should sit at 90° (as indicated by the diagram).

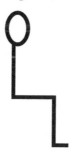

6   Ensure that you are lying down.

7   Ensure that you are in the following position [specify].

8   If someone is helping you with meals or drinks, make sure you are both at the same level so you can enjoy good eye contact and are able to maintain your posture.

Comments

Routledge
Taylor & Francis Group

Verbal Prompts

Note: Verbal prompts help to remind and draw the individual's attention to when and how to swallow.

1   You need verbal directions, using agreed vocabulary that you both understand. These directions should be short and to the point. Long sentences should not be used.

2   Avoid talking while chewing or swallowing.

Comments

Tactile Prompts

Note: Tactile prompts help to remind and draw the individual's attention to when and how to swallow.

1   You will need gentle verbal, non-verbal or physical prompts to sit down.

2   Have one item at a time on your [plate / bowl].

3   You need food or drink placed within your visual field.

4   To emphasise and encourage visual and tactile interaction, touch the mealtime equipment when you are about to use it.

5   You need utensils to be placed in your hand at the start of the meal and, if necessary, each time you put them down, until you have finished eating or drinking.

6   You should have your arm guided to pick up cutlery.

7   You should have hand-over-hand guidance to load or use utensils.

8   You should have your hand or arm guided to pick up food or drink, or for the food or drink to be placed in your hand. You may need prompts to take food to your mouth.

9   Touch the lips with the [mealtime equipment] [food] to encourage mouth opening.

10 Hold the [cup / straw / teat] until you have finished drinking.

11 Have food and drinks alternately.

12 Ensure that each course is kept at the correct temperature [specify] and served when ready to be eaten.

14 Have larger mouthfuls to stimulate jaw movement and control.

> **Comments**
>
>
>

Lip, Jaw and Head Support

1 The person who is helping you with meals or drinks needs to stand behind you to ensure that he or she can give the appropriate head support that you need. A mirror allows you to see each other in order to communicate.

2 The person who is helping you with meals or drinks should use hand support to assist you with jaw and lip closure (as shown in the diagram).

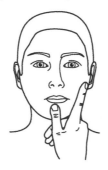

3 The person who is helping you with meals or drinks should use hand support to assist you with jaw closure (as shown in the diagram).

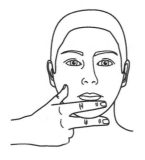

Routledge
Taylor & Francis Group
ROUTLEDGE

4   The person who is helping you with meals or drinks should use hand support to assist you with lip closure (as shown in the diagram).

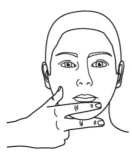

5   The person who is helping you with meals or drinks should support you as indicated in the diagram.

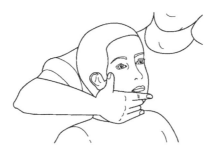

Comments

EATING AND DRINKING ADVICE DURING SWALLOWING

Note: The following techniques should be implemented whenever you are eating and drinking the foods or drinks specified in the 'Texture and consistencies' section.

1   Please complete 'Drink and Mealtime Diary Sheets' for ____ days.

2   Attempt to hold cutlery and cups yourself in order to maximise your independence and to prompt a better swallow.

3   If you are unable to feed yourself, you should hold the cutlery and crockery as best as you can, whilst someone else helps you to guide the food or drink. This will prompt a better swallow.

Routledge
Taylor & Francis Group

4 You need to be told what the food is and when it is approaching your mouth.

5 Take small-sized mouthfuls.

6 Take large-sized mouthfuls.

7 The spoon should be placed in the front of your mouth to allow you to draw off the food with your lips.

8 Maintain cup and lip contact between sips.

9 You should be encouraged to stabilise the cup by allowing it to rest on your lower teeth.

10 [Before / Once] the food or fluid is in the mouth stroke the individual's top lip down from the nose to the top lip to help lip closure.

11 Place food into the [front / back] [left side / right side] of the mouth.

12 Press back and down onto the tongue with the spoon or fork to help food to the back of the mouth.

13 Place food on the biting surfaces of the teeth in order to stimulate chewing.

14 Place food or fluid under your tongue, then close your lips and swallow.

15 Place food onto the side of the tongue to improve its manipulation.

16 Place foods that need to be bitten (eg, sandwiches or biscuits) between the front teeth and press up under the chin until a small piece has been bitten off.

17 Tap the cheeks just in front of the ear lobes to encourage jaw closure.

18 Take your time as rushing and gulping food down will lead to more problems.

19 After [specify number] sucks, remove teat from the mouth.

20 Don't talk and chew or swallow at the same time.

21 Stimulate the swallow by firmly stroking down from under the chin past the Adam's apple (as shown in the diagram).

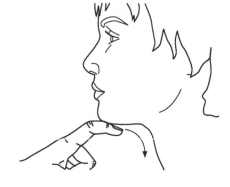

This page may be photocopied for instructional use only. *Swallowing Guidelines* © Elizabeth Boaden & Jo Walker, 2005

Routledge
Taylor & Francis Group

22 Take alternate swallows of food then a drink to help 'wash the food down'.

23 After each swallow, take two 'saliva-clearing swallows' to help to clear the residue from your throat.

24 Have the first mouthful of food or drink and then see if you can continue on your own.

25 Ensure that each mouthful has been swallowed before the next is taken.

26 You need to go at your own speed, not that of others.

27 Check for food pocketing in the cheeks and the roof of the mouth at regular intervals throughout the meal and when the meal is finished.

28 Cough or clear your throat if anything feels stuck or feels as if it has gone 'the wrong way'. Coughing or choking is your body's way of removing food or drink that may be stuck in the crevices in your throat, which may go into your lungs rather than into your stomach.

29 Pause for 2-3 minutes between courses.

30 If you get up from the table, or stop eating, you may not have finished and may need gentle prompts to complete your food or drink.

31 Make sure that you stay sitting up for at least 30 minutes after you have had something to eat or drink.

32 Clear around your mouth with your tongue or finger after meals.

33 After meals or drinks, sleep with the head of the bed raised to 30°.

34 To overcome your difficulties, ensure that when you swallow you [use a combination of the following]:

(a) Keep your head positioned centrally, looking forward while you are lying on your [right / left] side.

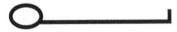

(b) Use a chin tuck (chin to chest while keeping your back straight). Hold this head posture before and while you swallow what is in your mouth.

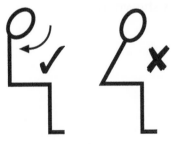

(c) Tip your head back [then swallow what is in your mouth].

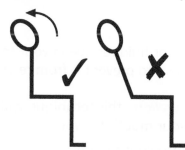

(d) Without moving your shoulders, turn your head to the [right/left] side so that your chin is over your shoulder. [Then swallow what is in your mouth.]

Right   Left

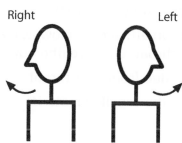

(e) Without moving your shoulders, tilt your head to the [right/left] side so that your ear nearly touches your shoulder. [Then swallow what is in your mouth.]

Right   Left

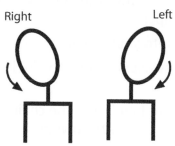

35 *Effortful swallow:* this will help the weak throat muscles to squeeze harder to prevent or remove residue in your throat. Each time you swallow; squeeze very hard with your tongue and throat. If you still have some food or fluid residue in your throat it is important to either spit it out or to swallow it to prevent it from re-entering your windpipe.

36 *Supra-glottic swallow:* this technique will help to co-ordinate your muscles to close off your windpipe before you swallow, ensuring all the food or drink goes down to your stomach:

- Put the food or drink into your mouth
- Once it is ready to be swallowed breathe in and let a little air out
- Hold your breath
- Swallow whilst still holding your breath
- Cough

Routledge
Taylor & Francis Group

- Swallow again to clear the expelled material
- Breathe normally.

If you still have some food or fluid residue in your throat, it is important either to spit it out or to swallow it to prevent it from re-entering your windpipe.

37 *Extended supra-glottic swallow:* this technique will help to transfer the food or drink to the back of your mouth for you to swallow:
- Put the food or fluid into your mouth
- Once it is ready to be swallowed, breathe in and let a little air out. Hold your breath and tip your head back so that all of the food or fluid in your mouth is now 'dumped' into your throat
- Continue to hold your breath and swallow as many times as you need to, in order to clear your throat, then breathe out
- Cough to clear any residue from your throat
- Swallow again to clear the expelled material
- Breathe normally.

If you still have some food or fluid residue in your throat, it is important either to spit it out or to swallow it to prevent it from re-entering your windpipe.

38 *Super supra-glottic swallow:* this technique will help to prevent food and fluid entering the windpipe:
- Put the food or drink into your mouth
- Once it is ready to be swallowed, breathe in, let a little air out and hold your breath
- Bear down, pushing your hands into the chair, and squeeze the muscles in your tongue and throat while swallowing
- Cough to clear any residue from your throat
- Swallow again to clear the expelled material
- Breathe normally.

If you still have some food or fluid residue in your throat, it is important either to spit it out or to swallow it to prevent it from re-entering your windpipe.

39 *Mendlesohn manoeuvre:* this technique will allow the muscle at the top of your food pipe to open wider, and for longer, preventing food and drink from becoming 'held up' in the throat:
- Put the food or drink into your mouth
- Once it is ready to be swallowed breathe in, let a little air out and start to swallow

- At the top of the swallow (when the Adam's apple is at its highest), use the muscles in the throat to hold it there for a few seconds.
- Once everything has been swallowed, let the tension go as you breathe out.

If you still have some food or fluid residue in your throat, it is important either to spit it out or to swallow it to prevent it from re-entering your windpipe.

40 *Suck-swallow:* this will increase the speed of initiation of the swallow. Pretend to suck something up a straw for several seconds then swallow the food or fluid that is in your mouth.

41 *Push/pull techniques:* these will help the voice box to close more effectively, and therefore will help to keep any food or drink from entering the windpipe. While you have food or drink held in your mouth, push or pull against a fixed object, then swallow what is in your mouth.

42 *Thermal stimulation:* when done before swallowing, this technique sends messages to the brain encouraging the muscles used for swallowing to prepare:

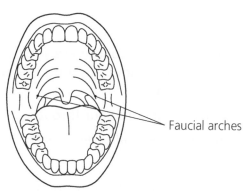

Faucial arches

- Dip the [specify] into cold water
- Then using a torch to see into the mouth, quickly rub both faucial arches (see diagram) downwards five times, holding the tongue down with a spatula
- Swallow a small amount of [saliva] [drink / food as specified in the 'Texture and consistencies' section]
- Repeat all steps before making further attempts at oral intake.

Comments

Swallowing Guidelines © Elizabeth Boaden & Jo Walker, 2005

Routledge
Taylor & Francis Group

COMPENSATORY TECHNIQUES TO PRACTICE

A   The following swallowing techniques are to be practised ＿＿ times a day.

B   Only swallow [your own saliva / the recommended consistency / sips of liquid / smooth semi-solids (eg, yoghurt or custard)].

C   On each practice session you should only swallow ＿＿ times/＿＿ mg/fl oz.

D   The following swallow techniques are only to be used [at breakfast / lunch / evening meals / snack times / during one meal a day / when you are having drinks / with saliva swallows].

1   *Effortful swallow*

This will help the weak throat muscles to squeeze harder to prevent or remove residue in your throat:

- Each time you swallow, squeeze very hard with your tongue and throat.

2   *Supra-glottic swallow*

This technique will help to coordinate your muscles to close off your windpipe before you swallow, ensuring that all the food or drink goes down to your stomach:

- Put the food or drink into your throat
- Once it is ready to be swallowed breathe in and let a litle air out
- Hold your breath
- Swallow whilst still holding your breath
- Cough
- Swallow again, to clear the expelled material
- Breathe normally

If you still have some food or fluid residue in your throat, it is important either to spit it out or to swallow it to prevent it from re-entering your windpipe.

3   *Extended supra-glottic swallow*

This technique will help to transfer food or drink to the back of your mouth for you to swallow:

- Put the food or fluid into your mouth.
- Once it is ready to be swallowed, breathe in and let a little air out. Hold your breath and tip your head back so all of the food or fluid in your

Routledge
Taylor & Francis Group

mouth is now 'dumped' in your throat

- Continue to hold your breath and swallow as many times as you need to in order to clear your throat
- Cough to clear any residue from your throat and then swallow again.

If you still have some food or fluid residue in your throat, it is important either to spit it out or to swallow it to prevent it from re-entering your windpipe.

4   *Super supra-glottic swallow*

This technique will help prevent food and fluid entering the windpipe:

- Put the food or drink into your mouth
- Once it is ready to be swallowed, breathe in, let a little air out and hold your breath
- Bear down, pushing your hands into the chair, and squeeze the muscles in your tongue and throat while swallowing
- Cough to clear any residue from your throat
- Swallow again to clear the expelled material
- Breathe normally.

If you still have some food or fluid residue in your throat, it is important either to spit it out or to swallow it to prevent it from re-entering your windpipe.

5   *Mendlesohn manoeuvre*

This technique will allow the muscle at the top of your food pipe to open wider and for longer, preventing food and drink becoming 'held up' in the throat:

- Put the food or drink into your mouth
- Once it is ready to be swallowed breathe in, let a little air out and start to swallow
- At the top of the swallow (when the Adam's apple is at its highest), use the muscles in the throat to hold it there for a few seconds.
- Once everything has been swallowed, let the tension go as you breathe out.

If you still have some food or fluid residue in your throat, it is important either to spit it out or to swallow it to prevent it from re-entering your windpipe.

This page may be photocopied for instructional use only. *Swallowing Guidelines* © Elizabeth Boaden & Jo Walker, 2005

Routledge
Taylor & Francis Group

6 *Thermal stimulation*

When done before swallowing, this technique sends messages to the brain encouraging the muscles used for swallowing to prepare.

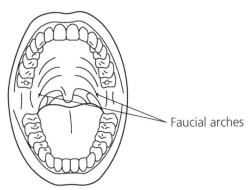

Faucial arches

- Dip the [specify] into cold water
- Then, using a torch to see into the mouth quickly rub both faucial arches (see diagram) downwards five times, holding the tongue down with a spatula
- Swallow
- Repeat all steps before further attempts to swallow.

> **Comments**

OROMOTOR THERAPY EXERCISES

These exercises will help to strengthen and increase the flexibility of muscles needed for chewing and swallowing, and should be done between mealtimes, that is, not with food or drink.

You may struggle at first to do these exercises, but it is similar doing any exercise. You need to build muscle strength, flexibility and stamina gradually.

Make sure you are in the same position as recommended for swallowing.

Routledge
Taylor & Francis Group

Lips

1 Encourage lip rounding and lip seal around tubing of progressively decreasing diameter. Place tubing between the lips so they can form a tight grip, hold this position and pressure for five seconds. Repeat ____ times.

2 Place a spatula between the lips and resist its withdrawal. Repeat ____ times.

3 Brush or tap around the outer lip region. Repeat ____ times.

4 Hold the lips together, initially for five seconds. Progress to 1–2 minutes. Repeat ____ times.

5 Close the lips tightly together, and whilst holding this position, gently suck in, causing the lips to be drawn in towards the mouth and increasing the pressure. Repeat ____ times.

6 Place the fingers on the cheeks and draw the lips forwards to encourage lip pouting. Repeat ____ times.

7 Stroke the top lip down from the tip of the nose to the lip. Repeat ____ times.

8 Keeping the lips together, blow air into the cheeks and then hold. Keep the cheeks puffed up, full of air. Do not allow air to escape from either the lips or nose. Repeat ____ times.

9 Smack the lips together slowly 10 times then repeat, this time doing 10 at a quicker rate. Repeat this whole sequence ____ times.

Comments

Routledge
Taylor & Francis Group

ROUTLEDGE

Tongue

1. Push your tongue out against a wet spatula, hold this stretch and pressure. Repeat ___ times.

2. Lift up your tongue tip against a wet spatula, hold this stretch and pressure. Repeat ___ times.

3. Push your tongue to the [left/right] against a wet spatula, hold this stretch and pressure. Repeat ___ times.

4. Hold a [liquorice stick / catheter tube / wrapped chewable material in gauze]. Place it onto the tongue and encourage lateral and circular tongue movements. Repeat ___ times.

5. Place a tiny amount of flavouring or sticky substance (eg, honey), behind the top teeth and lick it off with your tongue tip. Repeat ___ times.

6. With an open mouth position, lift the tongue tip up to the roof of the mouth, behind the front teeth. Hold this position and the pressure. Repeat ___ times.

7. Manipulate the [specify] around the mouth, and then bring it into a central position, between the tongue tip and the hard palate. This will encourage the tongue to cup the material. Then spit it out to prevent it being swallowed. Repeat ___ times.

8. Move [specify] around the mouth, and try to identify where in the mouth it is, for example front, back, sides, etc.

9. Using different-shaped sweets, for example Dolly Mixture™, without looking, try to identify which shape is in the mouth.

10. Use different tastes, temperatures, textured material and vibratory stimulation to improve sensation in the tongue.

11. Grip your tongue tip with your front teeth and swallow to improve the movement of the back part of the tongue and the muscles in the back of the mouth. Repeat ___ times.

12. Pretend to gargle. Repeat ___ times.

13. Pretend to yawn. Repeat ___ times.

14. Pull the back of the tongue into the back of the mouth, so that it forms a humped shape inside the mouth, and hold this position. Repeat ___ times.

15. Stick the tongue forward and out. Repeat ___ times.

Routledge
Taylor & Francis Group

16   Place a thin strip of gauze, soaked in juice, along the centre of the tongue. Squeeze the juice out by lifting the tongue up against the roof of the mouth. The juice should be [spat out / swallowed]. You should be able to see the shape of the tongue action on the dry gauze. Repeat ___ times.

Comments

Jaw

1   Support the jaw (see diagram) to help with different degrees of jaw control.

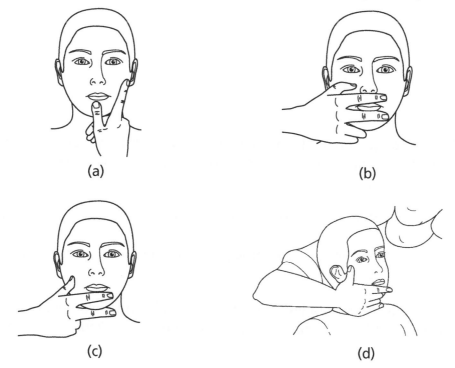

(a)

(b)

(c)

(d)

2   Stimulate the muscles that open and close the jaw by tapping and stroking each side of the jaw ___ times.

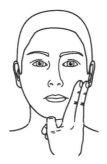

Routledge
Taylor & Francis Group

3   Wrap gauze around a chewable material (eg, pastille, fruit gum) and place on the back teeth. Ensure full lip closure and practise biting and chewing jaw movements, for ___ minutes.

4   Move the jaw from side to side, holding the position each time. Repeat this whole sequence ___ times.

5   Move the jaw in circular movements, as if chewing. Repeat ___ times.

6   Placing a thumb under the chin on the jaw bone, hold the jaw in a closed position whilst trying to open the jaw into an open-mouth position. Repeat ___ times.

Comments

Soft Palate

1   Hold your tongue tip gently between your teeth. Make a seal with your lips and blow out your cheeks with air. Hold this position and do not allow air to escape. Repeat ___ times.

2   Open the mouth wide and try to cause a yawn to occur. Repeat ___ times.

3   Say 'ah' five times, one after another, keeping the sound short, sharp and crisp. Repeat ___ times.

4   Using a straw, blow bubbles into a glass of water. This encourages all the air to come out of the mouth, rather than down the nose. Repeat ___ times.

Comments

Routledge
Taylor & Francis Group

Throat Muscles

1   Smoothly sing up the scale using the sound 'ah', and hold the highest note for 4-5 seconds. Repeat ___ times.

2   Lie on your back either on the floor or on the bed. Lift your head up so that you can see your toes, but don't lift your shoulders up. Hold for one minute, then rest for one minute. Repeat ___ times and ___ times each day.

3   Push or pull against a fixed object whilst saying 'ah'. Hold for ___ seconds. Repeat ___ times.

4   Take a breath, hold it tight for ___ seconds. Repeat ___ times.

Comments

This page may be photocopied for instructional use only. *Swallowing Guidelines* © Elizabeth Boaden & Jo Walker, 2005

Routledge
Taylor & Francis Group

Additional Resources

Tick for selection

☐ Drink and mealtime problem recording sheet

☐ Drink and mealtime problem diary sheet

☐ Label template

☐ Contact sheet

☐ Swallowing guidelines sign

Details

Routledge
Taylor & Francis Group
ROUTLEDGE

TEMPLATE
FOR SWALLOWING GUIDELINES

- Identify from the manual the statements and information applicable to the individual.

- Then circle the corresponding numbered statements and information on this templateto be included in the final programme and put a line through items or information to be deleted.

- Take care to write in specific additional information where indicated on this template.

Routledge
Taylor & Francis Group
ROUTLEDGE

SWALLOWING GUIDELINES

WRITTEN BY _____ **DATE** _____

NAME _____ **DOB** _____

Routledge
Taylor & Francis Group
ROUTLEDGE

DESCRIPTION OF SWALLOWING DIFFICULTIES

1   2

3   4

5   6

7   8

9 do exercises to strengthen muscles needed for swallowing

   practice how to swallow in a different way

   alter the way you swallow

   change the textures of what you eat and/or drink

Comments

ORAL DESENSITISATION EXERCISES

To be completed ____ times per day

1 lips / jaw;
   picture a b c d

2 Gently / Firmly   stroke / pat;
   repeat ____ times

3 Gently / Firmly   stroke / pat;
   repeat ____ times

4 Gently / Firmly stroke / pat;
   repeat ____ times

5 _____
   repeat ____ times

6 Gently / Firmly stroke / pat
   _____

7 Gently / Firmly;
   _____
   Repeat ____ times

8 _____
   Repeat ____ times

Routledge
Taylor & Francis Group

9   Gently / Firmly;

   10

_____

Repeat ___ times

11

> **Comments**
>
>
>
>
>
>
>

INTRODUCTION OF TOOTHBRUSH INTO THE MOUTH

To be completed ___ times per day

1   soft brush on little finger / small soft toothbrush / normal toothbrush;
Repeat ___ times

2   and repeat ___ times   3   and repeat ___ times

4   and repeat ___ times   5   and repeat ___ times

6

> **Comments**
>
>
>
>
>
>
>

Routledge
Taylor & Francis Group

ENVIRONMENT

1 a b c d e   2 a b c d

> **Comments**

EQUIPMENT

1   2 napkin / apron

3 meals   and   drinks, *your / a*

a	b ___	c ___	d ___	e ___
f ___	g ___	h ___	i ___	j ___
k ___	l ___	m ___	n ___	

> **Comments**

TEXTURE AND CONSISTENCIES

1 food / drink

Food

2 NV1   3 SE1

4 standard 7-month baby jars SD1   5 SC1

6 standard 4-month baby jars   7 SA1   SA2
   SB1   SB2

This page may be photocopied for instructional use only. *Swallowing Guidelines* © Elizabeth Boaden & Jo Walker, 2005

8   9   other examples _____

10   11

Drink

12   ND1   ND2   13

14   TD1   TD2   TD3   15   ___ scoops   SO1   SO2   SO3

16   ___ scoops   ST1   ST3   17   ___ scoops   S3

Medication

18   and thicken to ___ consistency   19

20

> **Comments**

GENERAL ADVICE AND PROMPTS

Note: You may want to change pronouns to direct the audience perspective, for example you to your child or to the client's name.

When to eat and drink

1   _____   2

3   4

5   6

> **Comments**

Preparation

1

2

3   so that you will be able to hear   4

Comments

Tracheostomy Guidelines

1   2

3   4

5   6

7   8

9   10

Comments

Routledge
Taylor & Francis Group

Positioning

1 support features, ie _____   2

3   4

5   6

7 _____   8

Comments

Verbal Prompts

1   2

Comments

Tactile Prompts

1   2 plate / bowl

3   4

5   6

7   8

9 mealtime equipment / food   10 cup / straw / teat

11   12

13

Comments

Lip, Jaw and Head Support

1   2

3   4

5

Comments

EATING AND DRINKING ADVICE DURING SWALLOWING

1 ____ days   2

3   4

5   6

7   8

9   10 Before / Once

11 front / back / left side /
     right side   12

 Routledge
Taylor & Francis Group

13
14

15
16

17
18

19
20

21
22

23
24

25
26

27
28

29
30

31
32

33
34 use a combination of the following:
a right / left;   b;
c then swallow;
d right / left   then swallow
right picture / left picture
e right / left   then swallow
right picture / left picture

35
36

37
38

39
40

41
42 saliva / drink / food

Comments

Routledge
Taylor & Francis Group

COMPENSATORY TECHNIQUES TO PRACTISE

A ___ times

B your saliva / recommended
   consistency / liquid / semi-solids

C ___ times, ___ mg / fl oz

D at breakfast / lunch / evening
   meals / snacks / x1 meal /
   drinks / saliva

1

2

3

4

5

6 _____

Comments

OROMOTOR THERAPY EXERCISES

Lips

1 ___ times   2 ___ times   3 ___ times

4 ___ times   5 ___ times   6 ___ times

7 ___ times   8 ___ times   9 ___ times

Comments

This page may be photocopied for instructional use only. Swallowing Guidelines © Elizabeth Boaden & Jo Walker, 2005

Routledge
Taylor & Francis Group

Tongue

1 ___ times

2 ___ times

3 right / left ___ times

4 liquorice / tube / _____ / gauze; ___ times

5 ___ times

6 ___ times

7 _____ ___ times

8 _____

9

10

11 ___ times

12 ___ times

13 ___ times

14 ___ times

15 ___ times

16 spat out / swallowed ___ times

Comments

Jaw

1 a b c d

2 ___ times

3 ___ minutes

4 ___ times

5 ___ times

6 ___ times

Comments

Routledge
Taylor & Francis Group
ROUTLEDGE

Soft Palate

1 ___ times

2 ___ times

3 ___ times

4 ___ times

Comments

Throat Muscles

1 ___ times

2 ___ times and ___ times each day

3 ___ seconds ___ times

4 ___ seconds ___ times

Comments

Routledge
Taylor & Francis Group
ROUTLEDGE

Additional Resources

Tick for selection

☐ Drink and mealtime problem recording sheet

☐ Drink and mealtime Problem diary sheet

☐ Label template

☐ Contact sheet

☐ Swallowing guideline signs

Details

Routledge
Taylor & Francis Group

ADDITIONAL RESOURCES

DRINK AND MEALTIME PROBLEM RECORDING SHEET

Identifying difficulties

Name _____ DOB _____

Date	Time	Type of food or drink	Describe the problem (if any) when getting food or drink into the mouth	Describe the problem, once drink is in the mouth	Describe the problem when food or drink is swallowed	Describe the problem after food or drink is swallowed

DRINK AND MEALTIME DIARY SHEET

Identifying quantity taken

Name _____ DOB _____

Date	Breakfast	Mid-morning	Lunchtime	Afternoon	Dinner	Supper	Other
	What had	What had	What had	What had	What had	What had	What had
	Amount taken Drinks Food	Amount taken Drinks Food	Amount taken Drinks Food	Amount taken Drinks Food	Amount taken Drinks Food	Amount taken Drinks Food	Amount taken Drinks Food
	What had	What had	What had	What had	What had	What had	What had
	Amount taken Drinks Food	Amount taken Drinks Food	Amount taken Drinks Food	Amount taken Drinks Food	Amount taken Drinks Food	Amount taken Drinks Food	Amount taken Drinks Food

Routledge
Taylor & Francis Group
ROUTLEDGE

SWALLOWING GUIDELINES SIGN

Name _____

Fluids			
ND	ND1	ND2	
TD	TD1	TD2	TD3
SO	SO1	SO2	SO3
ST	ST1		ST3
S			S3

Food			
NV	NV1		
SE	SE1		
SD	SD1		
SC	SC1		
SB	SB1	SB2	
SA	SA1	SA2	

Positions			
CTC	RTT	RTN	
HB	LHT	LHN	
(a)	(b)	(c)	
LD	(d)	U	

Additional information

Advised by _____ Date _____

Routledge
Taylor & Francis Group

ROUTLEDGE

DIAGRAMS FOR SWALLOWING GUIDELINE SIGNS

Insert any of the pictures below into the template provided to make a personalised sign. Alternatively, use the text boxes to write your own guidelines. Some examples can be seen in Appendix 1.

Fluids

Normal drinks **Examples:** water, tea, coffee, squash **ND**	**ND1**	**ND2**	
Naturally thick drinks; leaves a coating on empty glass. **Examples:** full-cream milk, supplement drinks **TD**	**TD1**	**TD2**	**TD3**
Thickened drinks Stage one: ____ scoops/200 ml Leaves thin coating on the back of a spoon **SO**	**SO1**	**SO2**	**SO3**
Thickened drinks Stage two: ____ scoops/200 ml Leaves a thick coating on the back of a spoon **ST**	**ST1**		**ST3**
Thickened drinks Stage three: ____ scoops/200 ml Needs to be taken by spoon **S**			**S3**

Routledge
Taylor & Francis Group

Food

Normal and varied diet ***Examples:*** meat, vegetables, biscuits. **NV**	**NV1**	
Soft moist foods (Stage E) ***Examples:*** tender meat casserole (1.5 cm diced pieces), mashed potato **SE**	**SE1**	
Mashed, moist, easy-chew foods (Stage D) ***Examples:*** flaked fish in sauce, stewed apple and thick custard **SD**	**SD1**	
Thick, smooth, uniform consistency – no chewing required (Stage C) ***Examples:*** mousse, blended mince and gravy **SC**	**SC1**	
Smooth, moist drop consistency (Stage B) ***Examples:*** thick custard, whipped cream **SB**	**SB1**	**SB2**
Smooth, pouring consistency (Stage A) ***Examples:*** creamed soup, thin custard **SA**	**SA1**	**SA2**

Routledge
Taylor & Francis Group

Positions

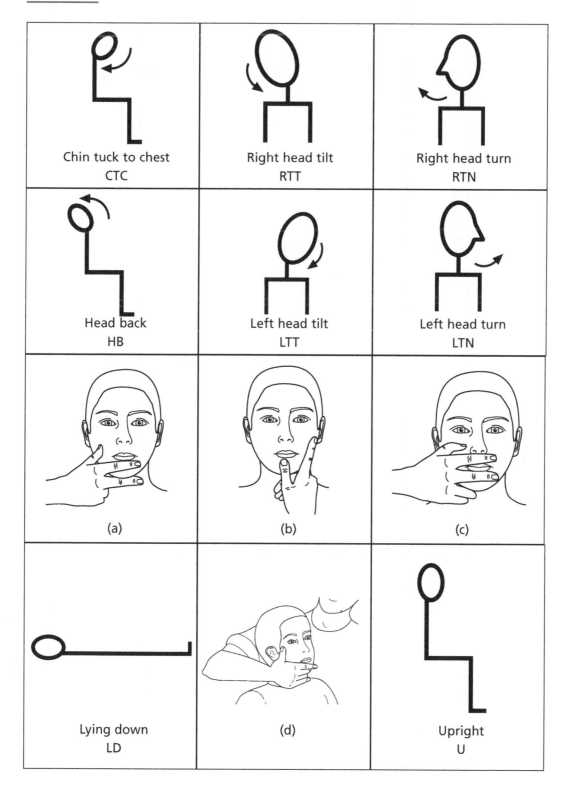

Chin tuck to chest
CTC

Right head tilt
RTT

Right head turn
RTN

Head back
HB

Left head tilt
LTT

Left head turn
LTN

(a)

(b)

(c)

Lying down
LD

(d)

Upright
U

Routledge
Taylor & Francis Group

SWALLOWING GUIDELINES

Name _____

DOB _____

Drinks

Food

Position

Additional information

Advised by _____

Date _____

LABEL TEMPLATE

A template of labels to be printed out. These can then be placed in drug charts, prescriptions, or on medication cabinets.

SWALLOWING DIFFICULTIES All medication to be given in syrup/soluble form	**SWALLOWING DIFFICULTIES** All medication to be given in syrup/soluble form	**SWALLOWING DIFFICULTIES** All medication to be given in syrup/soluble form
SWALLOWING DIFFICULTIES All medication to be given in syrup/soluble form	**SWALLOWING DIFFICULTIES** All medication to be given in syrup/soluble form	**SWALLOWING DIFFICULTIES** All medication to be given in syrup/soluble form
SWALLOWING DIFFICULTIES All medication to be given in syrup/soluble form	**SWALLOWING DIFFICULTIES** All medication to be given in syrup/soluble form	**SWALLOWING DIFFICULTIES** All medication to be given in syrup/soluble form
SWALLOWING DIFFICULTIES All medication to be given in syrup/soluble form	**SWALLOWING DIFFICULTIES** All medication to be given in syrup/soluble form	**SWALLOWING DIFFICULTIES** All medication to be given in syrup/soluble form
SWALLOWING DIFFICULTIES All medication to be given in syrup/soluble form	**SWALLOWING DIFFICULTIES** All medication to be given in syrup/soluble form	**SWALLOWING DIFFICULTIES** All medication to be given in syrup/soluble form

Routledge
Taylor & Francis Group

USEFUL CONTACTS

Routledge
Taylor & Francis Group
ROUTLEDGE

APPENDIXES

APPENDIX 1 EXAMPLES OF PROGRAMMES PRODUCED FOR EACH CLIENT GROUP

The following names and personal details are fictitious and are only used to demonstrate the use of this resource.

SWALLOWING GUIDELINES

WRITTEN BY _Mark Hill_   **DATE** _13.10.03_

NAME _Martin Dixon_   **DOB** _07.02.02_

DESCRIPTION OF SWALLOWING DIFFICULTIES

The throat muscles are not coordinating properly. This means that rather than food or drink going down your throat to the stomach, there is a risk of it going into the lungs. This is called 'aspiration'.

ORAL DESENSITISATION EXERCISES

- Firmly stroke the cheeks in preparation for oral desensitisation and repeat 5 times.

- Firmly stroke under the chin, jaw, cheeks and lips, working towards the mouth and repeat 3 times.

Routledge
Taylor & Francis Group

- Firmly stroke down the sides of the nose towards the upper lip (as indicated on the diagram) and repeat 3 times.

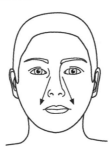

- Place a gloved, small wet finger, as an oral stimulator, underneath the top lip and slide it firmly and slowly along the upper gum.

  Repeat three times and then turn the oral stimulator so that the cheek is pushed out slightly.

  Pause, then repeat along the lower gum on the same side.

  Pause, then move the oral stimulator along gum on the opposite side.

  Pause, then move the oral stimulator along lower gum on the same side and repeat 3 times.

- Firmly stroke or pat the tongue tip with the gloved, small wet finger as an oral stimulator.

- Firmly move the gloved, small wet finger as an oral stimulator back towards the first third of the tongue and repeat 3 times.

- Use a gloved, small wet finger, as an oral stimulator, to press down on the tongue tip. Gradually move the pressure towards the back of the tongue (stop before gagging occurs) and move it forward again. Repeat 3 times, in time to music.

- Firmly place a gloved, small wet finger, as an oral stimulator, on the ridge behind the top teeth to indicate where to place the tongue tip.

- Encourage oral manipulation of textured objects.

- Encourage oral manipulation of objects that have been flavoured.

INTRODUCTION OF A TOOTHBRUSH INTO THE MOUTH

[To be completed 3 times/day.]

- Using a small headed soft toothbrush, rub along the outside of the upper and lower gum ridges, the biting surfaces of the teeth and the inside surface of the teeth and repeat 3 times.

Routledge
Taylor & Francis Group

- Brush the tongue, teeth and lips and repeat 3 times.

- Brush the sides of the tongue and repeat 3 times.

- Introduce tastes or toothpaste on the brush and repeat 3 times.

- Use an electronic toothbrush to introduce vibration into the mouth and repeat 3 times.

Comments

Martin's nutritional needs and fluid requirements are being met adequately via the tube. It is important to continue to do the exercises above in order to maintain oral sensation.

SWALLOWING GUIDELINES

WRITTEN BY _James Roberts_   **DATE** _09.04.04_

NAME _Rebecca Thomas_   **DOB** _26.01.87_

DESCRIPTION OF SWALLOWING DIFFICULTIES

- The messages being sent to and from the muscles in the mouth via the brain are damaged, causing the mouth to move in an uncoordinated or different way. It may be difficult to get food and drink into the mouth. Once it is in the mouth, the food and drink may then be difficult to control and may not be swallowed safely.

- Coughing is your body's natural way of removing material from your windpipe and is at times normal.

- When something does 'go down the wrong way' and into the lungs, this is called 'aspiration'. Signs of aspiration are: excessive or frequent coughing; wet, gargly voice quality; change in breathing rate; change in colour; recurrent chest infections. If aspiration occurs frequently it can cause chronic chest infections and problems. This may mean that you need to: do exercises to strengthen muscles needed for swallowing; practice how to swallow in a different way; alter the way you swallow; change the textures of what you eat and/or drink. It is important to follow the guidelines below to prevent or reduce the severity of the swallowing problem, and to minimise the risk of choking or swallowing things the wrong way. If any difficulties are noted, please check that the advice is being followed, before contacting the person identified on the front of the guidelines.

Routledge
Taylor & Francis Group
ROUTLEDGE

ENVIRONMENT

Note: The environment affects muscle tone and influences individuals' ability to concentrate and to swallow.

If it helps, eat in a more stimulating environment. Consider:

- brightly coloured mats or cutlery
- sitting at a table with others in a small group.

EQUIPMENT

Note: Special equipment may improve the way in which food and drink is received.

For meals and drinks check that you are using a:

- dysphagia cup
- special angled cutlery
- non-slip mat

TEXTURES AND CONSISTENCIES

Note: Some consistencies are easier and safer to swallow than others.

You should have foods that are soft and moist, for example tender meat casseroles (approx 1.5 cm-diced pieces), mashed potato, sponge and custard. Avoid foods:

- of a mixed consistency, such as cereals that do not absorb milk;
- that are hard and dry, such as nuts, pastry and biscuits;
- which have husks, skins or are fibrous, such as sweetcorn, peas, grapes, beans, celery and orange.

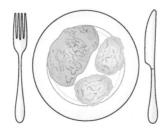

This page may be photocopied for instructional use only. *Swallowing Guidelines* © Elizabeth Boaden & Jo Walker, 2005

Routledge
Taylor & Francis Group
ROUTLEDGE

You should have drinks that are naturally thicker in consistency, for example full cream milk, supplement drinks or sip feeds.

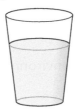

Medication

- Ensure that all tablets are taken with a drink that is of the specified consistency.

GENERAL ADVICE AND PROMPTS

When to eat and drink

Note: The throat muscles may tire at specific times of the day, or during the meal, which may cause aspiration or inadequate nutrition.

- Meals should be spaced out evenly throughout the day.

- Since one tires as the day goes on, make sure that you are having a large meal and frequent drinks at the start of the day and just light snacks later.

Positioning

Note: Posture affects both muscle tone and the ability to swallow.

- Use the recommended positioning equipment: that is, standing frame, wedges or wheelchair, and ensure that all the support features are secure, ie, headrest

- If someone is helping you with meals or drinks, make sure you are both at the same level so you can enjoy good eye contact and are able to maintain your posture.

> **Comments**
>
> Ensure that Rebecca has a small wedge placed in the small of her back, allowing her to lean slightly forwards at mealtimes with her elbows resting on her table.

 Routledge
Taylor & Francis Group

Verbal Prompts

Note: Verbal prompts help to remind and draw the individual's attention to when and how to swallow.

- You need verbal directions, using agreed vocabulary that you both understand. These directions should be short and to the point. Long sentences should not be used.

Tactile Prompts

Note: Tactile prompts help to remind and draw the individual's attention to when and how to swallow.

- You should have your arm guided to pick up cutlery.

- You should have hand-over-hand guidance to load or use utensils.

- Touch the lips with the mealtime equipment to encourage mouth opening.

Lip, Jaw and Head Support

- The person who is helping you with meals or drinks should use hand support to assist you with jaw and lip closure (as shown in the diagram).

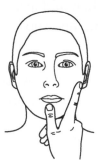

EATING AND DRINKING ADVICE DURING SWALLOWING

Note: The following techniques should be implemented whenever you are eating and drinking the foods or drinks specified in the 'Texture and consistencies' section.

- If you are unable to feed yourself, you should hold the cutlery and crockery as best as you can, whilst someone else helps you to guide the food or drink. This will prompt a better swallow.

- You need to be told what the food is and when it is approaching your mouth.

- Take small-sized mouthfuls.

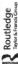

- The spoon should be placed in the front of your mouth to allow you to draw off the food with your lips.

- Maintain cup and lip contact between sips.

- You should be encouraged to stabilise the cup by allowing it to rest on your lower teeth.

- Place foods that need to be bitten (eg, sandwiches or biscuits) between the front teeth and press up under the chin until a small piece has been bitten off.

- Take alternate swallows of food then a drink to help 'wash the food down'.

- Pause for 2-3 minutes between courses.

- Make sure that you stay sitting up for at least 30 minutes after you have had something to eat or drink.

OROMOTOR THERAPY EXERCISES

These exercises will help to strengthen and increase the flexibility of muscles needed for chewing and swallowing, and should be done between mealtimes, that is, not with food or drink.

You may struggle at first to do these exercises, but it is similar doing any exercise. You need to build muscle strength, flexibility and stamina gradually.

Make sure you are in the same position as recommended for swallowing.

Lips

- Encourage lip rounding and lip seal around tubing of progressively decreasing diameter. Place tubing between the lips so they can form a tight grip, hold this position and pressure for five seconds. Repeat 5 times.

- Place a spatula between the lips and resist its withdrawal. Repeat 5 times.

Routledge
Taylor & Francis Group

Jaw

1   Support the jaw (see diagram) to help with different degrees of jaw control.

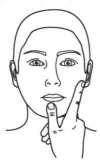

2   Stimulate the muscles that open and close the jaw by tapping and stroking each side of the jaw 5 times.

3   Wrap gauze around a chewable material (eg, pastille, fruit gum) and place on the back teeth. Ensure full lip closure and practise biting and chewing jaw movements, for 5 minutes.

Routledge
Taylor & Francis Group

SWALLOWING GUIDELINES

WRITTEN BY _Sarah Platt_   **DATE** _22.04.04_

NAME _David Tickle_   **DOB** _15.09.22_

DESCRIPTION OF SWALLOWING DIFFICULTIES

- The muscle in your throat, which opens and closes to control how and when food and drink are pushed down towards your stomach, is not opening in the right way and at the right time. Food and drink may enter the lungs instead of going down into the stomach. It may also cause a sticking sensation and may take many swallows to get a very small quantity of food and drink down. This can be extremely tiring.

- When something does 'go down the wrong way' and into the lungs, this is called 'aspiration'. Signs of aspiration are: excessive or frequent coughing; wet, gargly voice quality; change in breathing rate; change in colour; recurrent chest infections. If aspiration occurs frequently it can cause chronic chest infections and problems. This may mean that you need to: do exercises to strengthen muscles needed for swallowing; practice how to swallow in a different way; alter the way you swallow; change the textures of what you eat and/or drink. It is important to follow the guidelines below to prevent or reduce the severity of the swallowing problem, and to minimise the risk of choking or swallowing things the wrong way. If any difficulties are noted, please check that the advice is being followed, before contacting the person identified on the front of the guidelines.

ENVIRONMENT

Note: The environment affects muscle tone and influences individuals' ability to concentrate and to swallow.

If it helps, eat in a quiet room without too many distractions. Consider:

- moving away from people who are talking or moving around, as this may be distracting

 Routledge
Taylor & Francis Group

EQUIPMENT

Note: Special equipment may improve the way in which food and drink is received.

For meals check that you are using a:

- plate guard
- insulated bowl
- non-slip mat

TEXTURES AND CONSISTENCIES

Note: Some consistencies are easier and safer to swallow than others.

- You should have foods that are smooth and moist with a 'drop' consistency. This texture would slip through a fork and needs to be eaten with a spoon, for example thick custard or soft whipped cream.

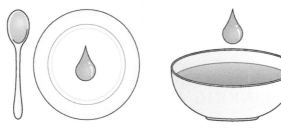

- Using the thickener prescribed, thicken all thin fluids to a milky consistency. This texture can be drunk through a straw or cup but would leave a thin coating on the back of a spoon (approx 2 scoops of prescribed thickener per 200 ml). Please follow the manufacturer's instructions.

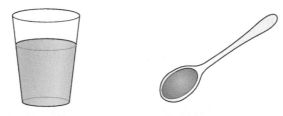

Medication

- All medication should be taken in syrup or soluble form.

Routledge
Taylor & Francis Group

GENERAL ADVICE AND PROMPTS

Positioning

Note: Posture affects both muscle tone and the ability to swallow.

- Make sure that you are close enough to the table.

- You should be able to reach your meal and drink comfortably.

- Your hips, body, shoulders and head should all be aligned, and you should sit at 90° (as indicated by the diagram).

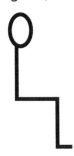

EATING AND DRINKING ADVICE DURING SWALLOWING

Note: The following techniques should be implemented whenever you are eating and drinking the foods or drinks specified in the 'Texture and consistencies' section.

- Please complete 'Drink and Mealtime Diary Sheets' for 7 days.

- Take small-sized mouthfuls.

- After each swallow, take two 'saliva-clearing swallows' to help to clear the residue from your throat.

- Ensure that each mouthful has been swallowed before the next is taken.

- You need to go at your own speed, not that of others.

- Cough or clear your throat if anything feels stuck or feels as if it has gone 'the wrong way'. Coughing or choking is your body's way of removing food or drink that may be stuck in the crevices in your throat, which may go into your lungs rather than into your stomach.

- Pause for 2-3 minutes between courses.

Routledge
Taylor & Francis Group
ROUTLEDGE

- Make sure that you stay sitting up for at least 30 minutes after you have had something to eat or drink.

- To overcome your difficulties, ensure that when you swallow you [use a combination of the following]:

  - Use a chin tuck (chin to chest while keeping your back straight). Hold this head posture before and while you swallow what is in your mouth.

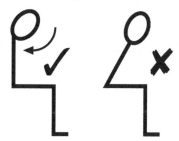

  - Without moving your shoulders, turn your head to the right side so that your chin is over your shoulder. Then swallow what is in your mouth.

Right

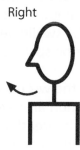

- *Mendlesohn manoeuvre:* this technique will allow the muscle at the top of your food pipe to open wider, and for longer, preventing food and drink from becoming 'held up' in the throat:

  - Put the food or drink into your mouth

  - Once it is ready to be swallowed breathe in, let a little air out and start to swallow

  - At the top of the swallow (when the Adam's apple is at its highest), use the muscles in the throat to hold it there for a few seconds.

  - Once everything has been swallowed, let the tension go as you breathe out.

  If you still have some food or fluid residue in your throat, it is important either to spit it out or to swallow it to prevent it from re-entering your windpipe.

Routledge
Taylor & Francis Group

SWALLOWING GUIDELINES

WRITTEN BY ___Jane Smith___   DATE ___27.09.03___

NAME ___Daniel Jones___   DOB ___04.12.38___

DESCRIPTION OF SWALLOWING DIFFICULTIES

- The messages being sent to and from the muscles of the mouth via the brain are damaged. Consequently, the mouth is not always able to detect that food or drink is present and needs to be swallowed. Overlarge bites may be taken, or food may stay in the mouth or be spat out.

- When something does 'go down the wrong way' and into the lungs, this is called 'aspiration'. Signs of aspiration are: excessive or frequent coughing; wet, gargly voice quality; change in breathing rate; change in colour; recurrent chest infections. If aspiration occurs frequently it can cause chronic chest infections and problems. This may mean that you need to: do exercises to strengthen muscles needed for swallowing; practice how to swallow in a different way; alter the way you swallow; change the textures of what you eat and/or drink. It is important to follow the guidelines below to prevent or reduce the severity of the swallowing problem, and to minimise the risk of choking or swallowing things the wrong way. If any difficulties are noted, please check that the advice is being followed, before contacting the person identified on the front of the guidelines.

ENVIRONMENT

Note: The environment affects muscle tone and influences individuals' ability to concentrate and to swallow.

If it helps, eat in a quiet room without too many distractions. Consider:

- reducing background noise (eg, turn off radio or television)
- moving away from people who are talking or moving around, as this may be distracting
- removing unnecessary things from the dining table (eg, flowers or tissues).

Routledge
Taylor & Francis Group
ROUTLEDGE

EQUIPMENT

Note: Special equipment may improve the way in which food and drink is received.

- Remember to use a napkin when eating and drinking.

> **Comments**
>
> *For meals, check that you are using your teaspoon.*

TEXTURES AND CONSISTENCIES

Note: Some consistencies are easier and safer to swallow than others.

- You should have foods that are soft, moist and easy to chew, for example Weetabix™, porridge, shepherd's pie, flaked fish in thick sauce, stewed fruit and thick custard.

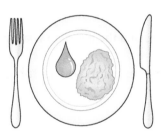

- You should have drinks that are naturally thicker in consistency, for example full cream milk, supplement drinks or sip feeds.

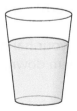

GENERAL ADVICE AND PROMPTS

When to eat and drink

Note: The throat muscles may tire at specific times of the day, or during the meal, which may cause aspiration or inadequate nutrition.

- Rather than having large meals, three times a day, try having smaller more frequent meals, Include snacks mid-morning, afternoon and suppertime.

Preparation

Note: It is important to be comfortable in order to concentrate and to be able to eat and drink as much of the meal as possible.

- Only eat when you are fully awake and alert.

- Make sure your glasses are clean, fit securely and are available at mealtimes.

- If you wear dentures for mealtimes, make sure that they fit and are fixed securely.

Positioning

Note: Posture affects both muscle tone and the ability to swallow.

- Make sure that you are close enough to the table.

Tactile Prompts

Note: Tactile prompts help to remind and draw the individual's attention to when and how to swallow.

- You will need gentle verbal, non-verbal or physical prompts to sit down.

- You need utensils to be placed in your hand at the start of the meal and, if necessary, each time you put them down, until you have finished eating or drinking.

- Ensure that each course is kept at the correct temperature, 75 degrees, and served when ready to be eaten.

Routledge
Taylor & Francis Group

EATING AND DRINKING ADVICE DURING SWALLOWING

Note: The following techniques should be implemented whenever you are eating and drinking the foods or drinks specified in the 'Texture and consistencies' section.

- Please complete 'Drink and Mealtime Diary Sheets' for 7 days.

- Check for food pocketing in the cheeks and the roof of the mouth at regular intervals throughout the meal and when the meal is finished.

- Cough or clear your throat if anything feels stuck or feels as if it has gone 'the wrong way'. Coughing or choking is your body's way of removing food or drink that may be stuck in the crevices in your throat, which may go into your lungs rather than into your stomach.

- Make sure that you stay sitting up for at least 30 minutes after you have had something to eat or drink.

Comments

Make sure you do not overload your mouth with food. Use the teaspoon to help control the amount you put in your mouth

---

Routledge
Taylor & Francis Group

USEFUL CONTACTS

Jane Smith
Speech and Language Therapist

0193 781 226

Sally Shaw
Dietician

0193 782 133

Kevin Wright
Key worker at day centre

0193 765 491

APPENDIX 2: DRINK AND MEALTIME PROBLEM RECORDING SHEET

Identifying difficulties

Name ___John Smith___   DOB ___15/11/63___

Date	Time	Type of food or drink	Describe the problem (if any) when getting food or drink into the mouth	Describe the problem, once drink is in the mouth	Describe the problem when food or drink is swallowed	Describe the problem after food or drink is swallowed
17/8/03	5.45pm	Peas				Coughing
17/8/03	6.15pm	Coffee	Drink running from cup and mouth down chin		Coffee squirting out between lips as swallowing	Some coughing after each swallow
19/8/03	8am	Milky tea	As above		Some escape from lips as swallow occurring	Becoming short of breath and coughing at end of drink
19/8/03	8.30am	Bran flakes			Trying to stifle coughing	Explosive coughing several times

Routledge
Taylor & Francis Group
ROUTLEDGE

APPENDIX 3: DRINK AND MEALTIME DIARY SHEET

Identifying quantity taken

Name ___Jane Thompson___   DOB _23.01.74_

Date	Breakfast	Mid-morning	Lunchtime	Afternoon	Dinner	Supper	Other
7/3/03	**What had** 1 weetabix tea **Amount taken** Drinks 200mls Food weetabix	**What had** nil **Amount taken** Drinks Food	**What had** Soup, tea **Amount taken** Drinks 150mls Food 250g	**What had** tea **Amount taken** Drinks 150mls Food	**What had** Fish pie, potato, yoghurt **Amount taken** Drinks Food ½ of all meal	**What had** Hot chocolate **Amount taken** Drinks 200mls Food	**What had** **Amount taken** Drinks Food
	What had 1 weetabix **Amount taken** Drinks 75mls Food 2 scrambled eggs	**What had** coffee orange juice **Amount taken** Drinks 100mls Food	**What had** 2 boiled eggs **Amount taken** Drinks 100mls Food 1 egg, yoghurt	**What had** tea tea, yoghurt **Amount taken** Drinks 75mls Food	**What had** cottage pie **Amount taken** Drinks 150mls Food ½ of all meal	**What had** Malt drink Trifle, tea **Amount taken** Drinks 175mls Food	**What had** **Amount taken** Drinks Food

APPENDIX 4: SWALLOWING GUIDELINES

Name ___Julie Lloyd___   DOB ___4/12/34___

Drinks
Thickened drinks, stage one: 1½ scoops/200 ml.
Leaves thin coating on the back of a spoon.

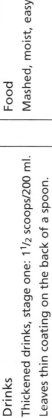

Food
Mashed, moist, easy-chew foods (Stage D)

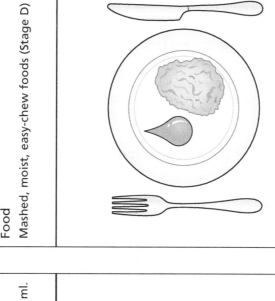

Position
Chin tuck to chest (CTC)

Additional information
Please ensure Mrs Lloyd is wearing her glasses

Advised by ___Jane Fisher___   Date ___2/10/05___

Routledge
Taylor & Francis Group
ROUTLEDGE

BIBLIOGRAPHY

Boylston E & O'Day C, 1999, *Successful Eating Dementia Swallowing Assessment*, Imaginart International Inc, Brisbee.

British Dietetic Association & Royal College of Speech and Language Therapists, 2002, *National Descriptors for Texture Modification in Adults,* BDA/RCSLT, London.

Chadwick DD, Joliffe J & Goldbart J, 2002, 'Carer Knowledge of Dysphagia Management Strategies', *International Journal of Language and Communication Disorders* 37(3), 345–57.

Cherney LR, 1994, *Clinical Management of Dysphagia in Adults and Children*, 2nd edn, Aspen Publishers Inc.

Dikeman KJ & Kazandjian MS, 1995, *Communication and Swallowing Management of Tracheostomized and Ventilator-Dependent Adults*, Singular Publishing Inc, San Diego.

Kindell J, 2002, *Feeding and Swallowing Disorders in Dementia,* Speechmark Publishing, Bicester.

Langley J, 1996, *Working with Swallowing Disorders,* Speechmark Publishing, Bicester.

Logemann J, 1993, *Manual for the Videofluorographic Study of Swallowing*, Pro-Ed Inc, Austin.

Marks L & Rainbow D, 2001, *Working with Dysphagia*, Speechmark Publishing, Bicester.

Morris SE & Klein MD, 2000, *Pre-Feeding Skills: A Comprehensive Resource for Feeding Development*, 2nd edn, Therapy Skill Builders, AZ.

Perlman AL & Schulze-Delrieu K, 1997, *Deglutition and Its Disorders: Anatomy, Physiology, Clinical Diagnosis and Management*, Singular Publishing Group Inc, San Diego.

Tipton Dikengil A, 1994, *Communication Carryover for Adults: Caregiver Information and Instruction*, The Psychological Corporation, London.

Veldee M & Miller R, 1992, *Handbook of Clinical Dietetics*, Yale University Press.

Winstock A, 1994, *The Practical Management of Eating & Drinking Difficulties in Children*, Speechmark Publishing, Bicester.

www.plainenglish.co.uk

Printed and bound by CPI Group (UK) Ltd, Croydon, CR0 4YY

17/10/2024

01775697-0019